CW01183891

Understanding Emotional Triggers

Understanding Emotional Triggers

Jennifer Carpenter

Copyright © 2025 by Jennifer Carpenter
All rights reserved. No part of this book may be reproduced in any manner whatsoever without written permission except in the case of brief quotations embodied in critical articles and reviews.
First Printing, 2025

Contents

1

Understanding Emotional Triggers

Defining Emotional Triggers

Defining emotional triggers is essential for anyone involved in the care of children, especially for surrogate parents, foster parents, and step-parents. Emotional triggers are specific stimuli—such as words, situations, or memories—that provoke strong emotional responses, often rooted in past experiences. Understanding these triggers is crucial for caregivers, as they can significantly impact interactions with children and influence the child's emotional development. By identifying these triggers, caregivers can create a more supportive and nurturing environment that fosters growth and resilience in children.

Recognizing emotional triggers begins with self-awareness. Caregivers must take the time to reflect on their own emotional responses and the underlying reasons for those feelings. This process can be enlightening, revealing patterns that might not have been previously acknowledged. For instance, a caregiver might notice that certain behaviors in a child evoke frustration or anxiety. By pinpointing these reactions, caregivers can work to mitigate their impact, allowing for more constructive interactions. This self-reflection is the first step toward building a healthier emotional landscape for both the caregiver and the child.

Once triggers are identified, caregivers can implement specific strategies to manage their emotional responses. Techniques such as mindfulness practices can be incredibly effective. Mindfulness encourages caregivers to stay present, allowing them to observe their emotions without immediate judgment or reaction. This practice can transform a potentially overwhelming emotional response into an opportunity for thoughtful engagement. As caregivers learn to pause and reflect before reacting, they model emotional regulation for the children in their care, reinforcing the importance of managing feelings in a constructive manner.

Building resilience in children is another vital aspect of understanding emotional triggers. When caregivers respond to triggers with awareness and compassion, they create a safe space for children to express their own emotions. This environment fosters emotional intelligence and resilience, equipping children with the tools they need to navigate their feelings. Caregivers can encourage this development by facilitating open conversations about emotions, helping children articulate their feelings, and validating their experiences. Such practices not only strengthen the caregiver-child bond but also empower children to develop healthy coping mechanisms.

Ultimately, the journey of defining and managing emotional triggers is a continuous process of growth for both caregivers and children. Training programs on emotional awareness can provide valuable resources and techniques for caregivers, enhancing their understanding and ability to navigate these challenges. Collaborative approaches between caregivers and parents can further enrich this learning, promoting a unified strategy for emotional development. By embracing this journey with an open heart and a willingness to grow, caregivers can create transformative experiences that lead to emotional healing and resilience for themselves and the children they nurture.

The Impact of Triggers on Caregiving

The emotional landscape of caregiving is often shaped by various triggers that can significantly impact how surrogate parents, foster parents, and step-parents navigate their roles. Understanding these triggers is essential for creating a nurturing environment for the children in their care. Triggers can stem from past experiences, emotional wounds, or even the behaviors of the children themselves. Recognizing these triggers not only helps caregivers manage their emotional responses but also fosters a more stable atmosphere for children, who may already be navigating their own challenges.

Developing effective strategies to manage emotional triggers is crucial for caregivers. This can involve setting aside time for self-reflection, journaling about emotional experiences, or engaging in open conversations with trusted friends or professionals. By identifying specific triggers and learning how to respond rather than react, caregivers can prevent their emotions from negatively influencing their caregiving. Creating a supportive network with other caregivers allows for sharing experiences and strategies, which can be incredibly validating and empowering.

Incorporating mindfulness practices into daily routines can further enhance emotional resilience for both caregivers and children. Mindfulness encourages present-moment awareness, which can help caregivers pause and reflect before responding to triggering situations. Simple breathing exercises, meditation, or even mindful walking can help caregivers ground themselves, reducing stress and promoting emotional balance. By modeling mindfulness, caregivers also teach children valuable coping skills that can serve them throughout their lives, reinforcing a sense of stability and security.

Building resilience in children is an essential aspect of caregiving that directly relates to managing emotional triggers. Caregivers can foster resilience by encouraging open communication, validating feelings, and promoting problem-solving skills. When children feel heard and understood, they are more likely to develop healthy coping mechanisms themselves. Engaging in collaborative techniques between caregivers and children—such as setting goals or creating action plans for challenging situations—can empower children to tackle difficulties with confidence, decreasing the likelihood of triggering emotional responses in caregivers.

Finally, training programs focused on emotional awareness can be instrumental for caregivers seeking to enhance their skills. These programs provide valuable insights into emotional triggers and effective coping strategies, equipping caregivers with the tools necessary for success. Whether through workshops, online courses, or community support groups, investing in education around emotional awareness fosters a culture of understanding and compassion in caregiving. As caregivers become more attuned to their emotional responses and the dynamics at play, they cultivate a nurturing environment that benefits both themselves and the children they care for.

Recognizing Your Own Triggers

Recognizing your own triggers is an essential step in fostering a nurturing environment for children in your care. As surrogate parents, foster parents, or step-parents, you are often faced with unique challenges that can evoke strong emotional responses. Understanding what triggers these reactions in yourself allows you to approach situations with greater awareness and control. It is not uncommon to feel overwhelmed or frustrated, especially when dealing with the complexities of a child's behavior. By identifying your triggers, you can create a foundation for emotional resilience that benefits both you and the children you support.

Begin by reflecting on moments when you feel your emotions intensifying. These instances might manifest as irritability, anxiety, or even sadness. Keeping a journal can be particularly helpful for tracking these feelings and identifying patterns over time. Note the specific situations, interactions, or words that elicit strong reactions. This practice not only aids in recognizing your triggers but also encourages you to articulate your emotions, making it easier to address them constructively. Over time, this self-awareness can help you respond to challenging situations with patience and understanding rather than frustration.

Mindfulness is a powerful tool for recognizing and managing your triggers. Taking a few moments each day to practice mindfulness techniques can enhance your emotional awareness. Simple breathing exercises, meditation, or even a short walk can help ground you and create mental space to observe your feelings without judgment. This practice fosters a sense of calm that can be invaluable when faced with challenging behaviors from the children in your care. By cultivating mindfulness, you equip yourself with the ability to pause, reflect, and choose your responses deliberately, promoting a more positive atmosphere for everyone involved.

Collaborative techniques can further support your journey in recognizing and addressing your triggers. Engaging in open dialogue with other caregivers or professionals can provide valuable insights and strategies. Sharing experiences not only normalizes the challenges you face but also empowers you to learn from others' coping mechanisms. Joining training programs focused on emotional awareness can deepen your understanding of triggers and develop practical skills for managing them effectively. This collaborative approach enriches your caregiving experience and creates a supportive network that benefits both you and the children in your care.

As you become more adept at recognizing your own triggers, you will notice a positive shift in your interactions with children. This growth fosters an environment where emotional resilience can flourish, not just for you, but for the children as well. By modeling self-awareness and proactive coping strategies, you teach children valuable lessons in emotional regulation and resilience. Remember, every step you take towards understanding your own triggers is a step towards creating a more harmonious and supportive home. Embrace this journey, and celebrate the progress you make, knowing that it will have a lasting impact on the lives of those you care for.

2

How to Move Past Psychological Triggers in Child C

Identifying Psychological Triggers

Identifying psychological triggers is a crucial step in fostering a nurturing environment for children in your care. As surrogate parents, foster parents, or step-parents, understanding what triggers specific emotional responses in both yourself and the children can significantly enhance your caregiving ability. Triggers can arise from various sources, such as past experiences, stressors in the present, or even certain words and actions that echo previous emotional wounds. By recognizing these triggers, you can not only manage your own reactions but also help children navigate their feelings, leading to healthier emotional responses.

To effectively identify psychological triggers, start by reflecting on your own emotional history. Consider moments when you felt overwhelmed or reactive; recognize the situations, people, or specific phrases that set off those feelings. Journaling can be particularly helpful in this process, allowing you to articulate your thoughts and feelings. This self-awareness will empower you to create a more stable emotional environment for the children you care for. Remember, fostering emotional intelligence in yourself lays the groundwork for teaching these skills to the children, promoting resilience and adaptability.

Children in your care may display behaviors that signal their own psychological triggers. Pay close attention to their reactions during various situations—do they withdraw, lash out, or become overly anxious? These responses can provide insight into their emotional landscape. Engaging in open, honest conversations with the children about their feelings can also reveal underlying triggers. Using age-appropriate language and encouraging them to express themselves helps build trust and opens the door for meaningful communication. This practice not only aids in identifying triggers but also cultivates an environment where children feel safe to explore their emotions.

Integrating mindfulness practices into your routine can greatly assist in identifying and managing triggers. Mindfulness encourages a present-focused awareness that can help both caregivers and children recognize emotional shifts before they escalate. Simple techniques, such as deep breathing or guided imagery, can provide grounding moments that allow you to pause and reflect before responding. Teaching these mindfulness techniques to children equips them with valuable tools to cope with their feelings, ultimately reducing the impact of their triggers over time.

As you cultivate your awareness of triggers, developing coping mechanisms becomes essential. Strategies such as positive reframing, where you consciously shift your perspective on a situation, can transform how you approach challenges. For children, creating a toolbox of coping strategies—like drawing, physical activity, or talking to a trusted adult—can empower them to manage their emotional responses. Training programs focused on emotional awareness for caregivers can further enhance these skills, creating a ripple effect of resilience and understanding within your caregiving dynamic. By working collaboratively with other caregivers and educators, you can share insights and techniques that promote emotional well-being for everyone involved.

Techniques for Reframing Triggers

Reframing triggers is a powerful technique that can transform the way caregivers respond to emotional challenges in child care. Understanding that triggers often stem from past experiences allows caregivers to approach these moments with a renewed perspective. Instead of feeling overwhelmed, surrogate parents, foster parents, and step-parents can view triggers as opportunities for growth and connection. By consciously choosing to reframe these emotional responses, caregivers can create a more supportive environment for themselves and the children in their care.

One effective method for reframing triggers involves identifying the specific emotions associated with a trigger. When a caregiver encounters a challenging behavior from a child, it is essential to pause and reflect on their feelings. By acknowledging emotions such as frustration, fear, or sadness, caregivers can begin to separate their reactions from the child's behavior. This awareness not only helps in managing their emotional responses but also sets a positive example for children on how to navigate their feelings. Over time, this practice cultivates resilience and emotional intelligence in both caregivers and children.

Mindfulness practices serve as a cornerstone for reframing triggers. Incorporating mindfulness techniques, such as deep breathing or grounding exercises, into daily routines allows caregivers to respond to triggers with a sense of calm. When faced with a stressful situation, taking a moment to focus on breathing can create a mental space for reflection rather than reaction. This shift in approach fosters a compassionate atmosphere, encouraging children to express their emotions without fear. Caregivers can also involve children in these practices, teaching them valuable skills to manage their own emotional triggers.

Another practical strategy for reframing triggers is to engage in collaborative discussions with children about emotions. Creating a safe space for open communication can empower children to articulate their feelings and experiences. Caregivers can guide these conversations by asking open-ended questions and encouraging children to share how certain situations make them feel. This collaborative approach not only strengthens the caregiver-child relationship but also builds emotional awareness and coping strategies in children. As caregivers model these discussions, they reinforce the idea that it is okay to explore and express one's feelings.

Finally, ongoing training and support are vital for caregivers seeking to enhance their ability to reframe triggers effectively. Participating in workshops or training programs focused on emotional awareness and resilience can equip caregivers with practical tools and techniques. These resources can provide caregivers with new perspectives on managing their emotional responses and understanding the triggers of the children they care for. By investing in their own emotional well-being and education, caregivers can create a nurturing environment that fosters growth and healing for themselves and the children they support.

Creating a Trigger-Response Plan

Creating a Trigger-Response Plan is an essential step for surrogate parents, foster parents, and stepparents navigating the emotional landscape of child care. Emotional triggers can arise unexpectedly, often leading to heightened stress for both caregivers and children. By developing a thoughtful and proactive plan, caregivers can better manage these triggers, fostering a nurturing environment that promotes healing and resilience. This plan will not only assist in recognizing triggers but also in formulating effective responses that support emotional growth for both the caregiver and the child.

The first step in creating a Trigger-Response Plan is identifying specific emotional triggers. Caregivers should take time to reflect on situations that lead to heightened emotional responses, whether those come from personal experiences or the child's behavior. Keeping a journal can be a beneficial strategy, allowing caregivers to document instances that evoke strong feelings. Over time, patterns may emerge, providing insight into both the caregiver's and the child's emotional landscape. Understanding these triggers is crucial for developing tailored strategies that address unique needs.

Once triggers are identified, caregivers can work on crafting appropriate response strategies. This involves defining how to react when confronted with these triggers, ensuring responses are grounded in mindfulness and emotional awareness. Techniques such as deep breathing, grounding exercises, or taking a moment of pause before responding can help caregivers manage their emotions effectively. Additionally, discussing these strategies with the child can help them understand the emotional dynamics at play, fostering an environment of open communication and mutual support.

Building resilience in children is an integral part of a Trigger-Response Plan. Caregivers should focus on teaching coping mechanisms that empower children to handle their own emotional triggers. Techniques such as role-playing, storytelling, or creative expression can be powerful tools for emotional regulation. Encouraging children to articulate their feelings and recognize their own triggers will foster both self-awareness and resilience. By equipping children with these skills, caregivers not only help them navigate their emotional challenges but also strengthen the caregiver-child bond.

Finally, collaboration with other caregivers and professionals can enhance the effectiveness of a Trigger-Response Plan. Engaging in training programs focused on emotional awareness can provide valuable insights and techniques that caregivers can implement. Networking with other parents and caregivers allows for the sharing of experiences and strategies, creating a supportive community. By working together, caregivers can cultivate an environment that prioritizes emotional health for both themselves and the children they care for, ultimately leading to more successful and fulfilling caregiving experiences.

3

Strategies to Manage Emotional Triggers

Emotional Regulation Techniques

Emotional regulation techniques are essential tools that caregivers can employ to navigate the often turbulent waters of child care. For surrogate parents, foster parents, and step-parents, understanding and mastering these techniques can make a significant difference in both their own emotional well-being and the emotional health of the children they care for. By learning to manage their own emotional triggers, caregivers can create a more stable and nurturing environment, fostering resilience and emotional growth in their children.

One effective technique for emotional regulation is mindfulness. Practicing mindfulness encourages caregivers to remain present and aware of their thoughts and feelings without judgment. This practice can be particularly beneficial in high-stress situations where emotional triggers may arise. By taking a moment to breathe deeply and center themselves, caregivers can cultivate a sense of calm and clarity, allowing them to respond to challenging behaviors with patience and understanding rather than reactivity. Incorporating mindfulness into daily routines, such as during mealtimes or bedtime, can also help establish a rhythm that promotes emotional stability for both caregivers and children.

Another powerful strategy is the use of positive self-talk. Caregivers often face daunting challenges that can induce feelings of inadequacy or frustration. By consciously reframing negative thoughts into positive affirmations, caregivers can shift their mindset and bolster their emotional resilience. For instance, replacing "I can't handle this" with "I am doing my best, and I will find a way through" helps cultivate a more optimistic outlook. This shift not only benefits the caregiver's emotional state but also sets a positive example for children, teaching them the importance of self-compassion and resilience.

Developing coping mechanisms is also crucial for caregivers working with children who may exhibit strong emotional responses. Identifying and implementing personalized coping strategies, such as journaling, engaging in physical activity, or seeking support from peers, empowers caregivers to manage their emotional states effectively. When caregivers take time to care for their own emotional needs, they are better equipped to support their children through challenging moments. This modeling of healthy coping can teach children valuable skills for their own emotional regulation, fostering resilience in them as they learn to navigate life's ups and downs.

Lastly, collaborative techniques can enhance emotional regulation for both caregivers and children. By fostering open communication and teamwork with children, caregivers can create a safe environment where feelings can be expressed and validated. Encouraging children to articulate their emotions not only helps them understand their own feelings but also strengthens the caregiver-child bond. Engaging in activities that promote teamwork, such as problem-solving tasks or group discussions about feelings, reinforces the idea that emotional experiences are shared and manageable. This collaborative approach not only aids in emotional regulation but also builds a strong foundation for trust and resilience within the family unit.

Establishing Healthy Boundaries

Establishing healthy boundaries is crucial for surrogate parents, foster parents, and step-parents who aim to create a nurturing and supportive environment for the children in their care. Healthy boundaries serve as a framework that not only protects your emotional well-being but also fosters a sense of security and stability for the children. When caregivers set clear limits on what is acceptable behavior, they create a safe space where children can explore their emotions and learn about relationships. This process requires careful reflection and a commitment to maintain those boundaries consistently.

To begin establishing healthy boundaries, caregivers should first assess their own emotional triggers. Understanding what situations or behaviors evoke strong emotional responses can guide you in defining your limits. By acknowledging your feelings, you can communicate your boundaries more effectively. For instance, if a child's behavior reminds you of a past trauma, recognizing this trigger allows you to respond thoughtfully rather than reactively. This self-awareness not only benefits your emotional health but also models emotional intelligence for the children, teaching them that recognizing and managing feelings is a vital life skill.

In addition to self-awareness, open communication is key to establishing boundaries. Engage in honest conversations with the children about what behaviors are acceptable and what are not. Use age-appropriate language to explain why certain boundaries are important and how they contribute to a positive living environment. Encourage children to express their feelings and concerns, reinforcing that their voices matter. This two-way communication fosters trust and respect, making it easier for children to understand and adhere to the boundaries you set.

Another effective strategy for maintaining healthy boundaries is to practice mindfulness. Mindfulness techniques, such as deep breathing or grounding exercises, can help caregivers stay calm and focused, especially during challenging situations. When caregivers model mindfulness, they not only manage their emotional triggers more effectively but also teach children valuable coping mechanisms. Incorporating regular mindfulness practices into your routine can enhance emotional resilience for both caregivers and children, making it easier to navigate the ups and downs of family dynamics.

Lastly, remember that setting and maintaining boundaries is an ongoing process that requires patience and flexibility. As relationships evolve, so too may your boundaries. Regularly revisiting and adjusting these boundaries ensures that they remain relevant and effective. Engaging in training programs focused on emotional awareness can equip you with additional tools and strategies to refine your approach. By committing to this journey, you not only enhance your well-being but also empower the children in your care to develop healthy relationship skills and emotional resilience that will serve them well throughout their lives.

Communication Strategies for Conflict Resolution

Effective communication is a cornerstone of conflict resolution, especially in the context of caregiving. Surrogate parents, foster parents, and step-parents often navigate complex emotional landscapes, not only for themselves but also for the children in their care. By adopting clear and empathetic communication strategies, caregivers can foster an environment of trust and understanding, which is crucial when addressing conflicts. Active listening is one of the most vital skills in this process; it involves fully engaging with the child's feelings and perspectives without interrupting or dismissing them. This practice not only validates their emotions but also opens the door to constructive dialogue.

Another essential communication strategy is the use of "I" statements. Rather than focusing on the child's behavior as the source of conflict, caregivers can express their feelings and needs directly. For example, instead of saying, "You never listen to me," a caregiver could say, "I feel frustrated when I am not heard." This approach encourages children to understand that their actions have an impact on others' emotions, promoting accountability while reducing defensiveness. By modeling this technique, caregivers not only address conflicts effectively but also teach children valuable emotional skills that they can carry into their future interactions.

Non-verbal communication also plays a significant role in resolving conflicts. Body language, facial expressions, and tone of voice can convey empathy and understanding, or they can escalate a situation if mismanaged. Caregivers should strive to maintain open and relaxed body language, ensuring that their non-verbal cues align with their verbal messages. This consistency helps to create a safe space where children feel secure enough to express their feelings. Mindfulness practices can aid caregivers in maintaining awareness of their own non-verbal signals, allowing for more intentional interactions that promote resolution rather than escalation.

In addition to these strategies, it is important to establish a routine for conflict resolution discussions. Setting aside regular times to check in with children about their feelings and any issues that may have arisen can prevent misunderstandings from festering. These discussions should be framed as opportunities for collaboration, where both the caregiver and the child can share their perspectives and work toward solutions together. This not only enhances the child's problem-solving skills but also reinforces the bond of trust between caregiver and child, making it easier to navigate future conflicts.

Finally, caregivers should remember the importance of patience and self-compassion throughout the conflict resolution process. Emotions can be intense, and progress may not always be linear. Celebrating small victories and acknowledging the efforts made by both the caregiver and the child can significantly enhance resilience and emotional growth. By remaining committed to open communication and practicing these strategies consistently, caregivers can create a nurturing environment that promotes healing, understanding, and lasting relationships.

4

Techniques for Building Resilience in Children

Understanding Resilience in Child Development

Understanding resilience in child development is a crucial aspect of nurturing emotionally healthy children, especially for surrogate parents, foster parents, and step-parents. Resilience refers to a child's ability to adapt positively in the face of adversity, challenges, or trauma. By fostering resilience, caregivers can help children develop the skills necessary to navigate life's ups and downs. Recognizing that children come with diverse backgrounds and experiences, it becomes essential to create an environment that encourages emotional growth and stability, allowing them to thrive despite obstacles.

One of the core components of resilience is the establishment of secure attachments. Children who feel safe and supported by their caregivers are more likely to develop the confidence to face challenges. As caregivers, it is vital to be consistently present, attentive, and responsive to a child's emotional needs. This can be achieved through active listening, validating their feelings, and providing reassurance. By building these secure attachments, caregivers lay the groundwork for resilience, helping children feel valued and understood in their unique situations.

Moreover, teaching children effective coping mechanisms is an integral part of building resilience. Caregivers can introduce strategies that empower children to manage their emotions in healthy ways. Techniques such as deep breathing, mindfulness, or journaling can help children express their feelings and reduce anxiety. Encouraging children to engage in problem-solving, rather than becoming overwhelmed by challenges, fosters a growth mindset. By modeling these behaviors and integrating them into daily routines, caregivers can significantly enhance a child's ability to cope with stress and setbacks.

Mindfulness practices also play a vital role in promoting resilience. When caregivers engage in mindfulness, they not only improve their emotional well-being but also set an example for the children in their care. Simple practices, such as guided meditation or nature walks, can help children learn to focus on the present moment and cultivate a sense of calm. These practices create a safe space for children to explore their feelings and develop emotional regulation skills. By incorporating mindfulness into everyday interactions, caregivers can help children build resilience while enhancing their emotional intelligence.

Lastly, collaboration among caregivers, educators, and mental health professionals is essential in fostering resilience within child development.

Training programs focused on emotional awareness can equip caregivers with the tools and strategies needed to support children effectively. By sharing experiences and techniques, caregivers can reinforce each other's efforts, creating a consistent and supportive environment for children. This collaborative approach not only strengthens the caregiver's ability to manage their emotional triggers but also promotes a holistic understanding of resilience, ultimately benefiting the children they care for.

Fostering Emotional Intelligence

Fostering emotional intelligence in children is a vital aspect of caregiving that can significantly influence their development and overall well-being. For surrogate parents, foster parents, and step-parents, understanding how to nurture emotional intelligence can help children navigate their feelings, build resilience, and form healthier relationships. By creating an environment that encourages emotional awareness, caregivers can empower children to recognize and express their emotions effectively. This process not only aids in the child's emotional growth but also fosters a deeper bond between the caregiver and the child.

One effective strategy for nurturing emotional intelligence is modeling emotional awareness. When caregivers openly express their feelings in appropriate ways, children learn to identify and label their own emotions. Sharing personal experiences related to emotions can help children understand that feeling a range of emotions is normal and acceptable. Caregivers can initiate discussions about their feelings during everyday situations, encouraging children to share their emotions without fear of judgment. This practice cultivates a safe space for emotional expression, laying the groundwork for children to develop their emotional vocabulary.

Incorporating mindfulness practices into daily routines can further enhance emotional intelligence. Mindfulness encourages both caregivers and children to be present in the moment and to acknowledge their feelings without judgment. Simple techniques such as deep breathing exercises, guided imagery, or mindful walking can help children learn to manage their emotions more effectively. By practicing mindfulness together, caregivers not only provide children with tools to cope with stress but also demonstrate the importance of self-regulation and awareness. This shared experience can strengthen the caregiver-child relationship, creating a foundation of trust and understanding.

Building resilience in children is another critical component of fostering emotional intelligence. Resilience enables children to bounce back from challenges and setbacks. Caregivers can support this by encouraging problem-solving skills and promoting a growth mindset. When children face difficulties, caregivers can guide them in reflecting on what they can learn from the experience, emphasizing that mistakes are opportunities for growth. Celebrating small successes and encouraging perseverance helps children develop confidence in their abilities, equipping them with the skills needed to handle future emotional triggers.

Lastly, collaborative techniques among caregivers, educators, and children can enhance emotional intelligence development. Engaging in open communication and sharing insights about children's emotional needs can create a unified approach to support their growth. Caregivers can participate in training programs focused on emotional awareness, enabling them to implement strategies that reinforce emotional intelligence at home and in educational settings. By working together and fostering an environment of support and understanding, caregivers can ensure that children feel valued and heard, ultimately nurturing their emotional well-being and resilience.

Encouraging Problem-Solving Skills

Encouraging problem-solving skills in children is a vital aspect of fostering resilience and emotional awareness, particularly for surrogate parents, foster parents, and step-parents. These caregivers often face unique challenges as they navigate the emotional complexities of the children in their care. By cultivating problem-solving abilities, caregivers empower children to tackle challenges independently, which can significantly reduce feelings of frustration and helplessness. This process begins with creating a supportive environment where children feel safe to express their thoughts and feelings, knowing that their caregivers are there to guide them through difficulties.

To effectively encourage problem-solving skills, caregivers can utilize open-ended questions that prompt critical thinking. Instead of providing immediate solutions to a child's problem, ask them how they might approach a situation or what alternatives they can think of. This technique not only fosters independence but also enhances a child's ability to evaluate options and make informed decisions. By engaging in this dialogue, caregivers demonstrate trust in the child's capabilities, reinforcing their self-esteem and encouraging them to take ownership of their problem-solving journey.

In addition to verbal encouragement, caregivers can introduce structured problem-solving activities. Simple tasks, such as puzzles or games that require strategic thinking, can be both enjoyable and educational. These activities help children learn to break down problems into manageable parts, assess possible solutions, and reflect on the outcomes of their decisions. Caregivers should celebrate the child's efforts and progress, regardless of the outcome, emphasizing that the learning process itself is valuable. This positive reinforcement nurtures a growth mindset, where children understand that mistakes are part of learning and can lead to greater resilience.

Mindfulness practices also play a crucial role in developing problem-solving skills. By integrating mindfulness techniques, such as deep breathing or visualization exercises, caregivers can help children manage their emotional triggers when faced with challenges. When children learn to pause and center themselves, they become more adept at assessing a situation calmly, which can lead to more thoughtful and effective problem-solving. Caregivers can model these practices, demonstrating how to approach problems with a clear mind and an open heart, thereby instilling these valuable techniques in the children they care for.

Ultimately, the journey of encouraging problem-solving skills is about fostering an environment where children feel empowered to face their fears and challenges head-on. As surrogate parents, foster parents, and step-parents, maintaining an encouraging tone and approach can significantly influence a child's emotional development. By equipping children with these essential skills, caregivers not only help them navigate current challenges but also prepare them for the complexities of life ahead. This commitment to nurturing problem-solving abilities will contribute to healthier emotional outcomes and a stronger bond between caregivers and children.

5

Mindfulness Practices for Child Care Providers

The Importance of Mindfulness in Caregiving

The practice of mindfulness is essential for caregivers navigating the complexities of surrogate, foster, and step-parenting. In the dynamic environment of caregiving, emotional triggers can arise unexpectedly, leading to reactions that may not reflect our true intentions. By embracing mindfulness, caregivers can cultivate a heightened awareness of their thoughts and emotions, enabling them to respond to challenging situations with clarity and compassion. This intentional focus helps in recognizing personal triggers, allowing caregivers to pause before reacting and choose a more constructive path.

Mindfulness equips caregivers with strategies to manage their emotional responses effectively. Techniques such as deep breathing, grounding exercises, and momentary pauses can be seamlessly integrated into daily routines, creating a space for reflection. These practices not only reduce stress but also foster a sense of calm that can positively influence the children in their care. As caregivers model these behaviors, they teach children valuable skills in emotional regulation, encouraging them to develop resilience in the face of adversity.

Building resilience in children is a fundamental aspect of caregiving that mindfulness can enhance. When caregivers approach challenging moments with a mindful mindset, they create an atmosphere of safety and understanding. This approach helps children feel seen and heard, allowing them to express their emotions without fear of judgment. By validating their feelings and guiding them through difficult emotions, caregivers can help children develop strong coping mechanisms that will serve them well into adulthood.

Training programs for educators on emotional awareness are increasingly recognizing the significance of mindfulness in caregiving. These programs not only equip caregivers with the tools to understand their emotional triggers but also emphasize the importance of self-care. Mindful practices such as meditation, journaling, or even simple moments of reflection can rejuvenate caregivers, allowing them to approach their responsibilities with renewed energy and perspective. The ripple effect of a caregiver's well-being directly impacts the emotional climate of the caregiving environment, promoting healthier relationships for everyone involved.

Collaboration among caregivers, whether they are surrogate parents, foster parents, or step-parents, is vital in nurturing a supportive community. Mindfulness encourages open communication, where caregivers can share their experiences, challenges, and coping strategies. This collaborative spirit not only fosters a sense of belonging but also empowers caregivers to learn from one another, enhancing their emotional awareness and resilience. Ultimately, embracing mindfulness in caregiving is a journey that not only benefits the caregivers themselves but also profoundly impacts the lives of the children they nurture.

Mindfulness Techniques for Daily Practice

Mindfulness techniques can significantly enhance the daily practice of surrogate, foster, and step-parents as they navigate the emotional landscape of caregiving. By integrating mindfulness into your routine, you can cultivate a sense of presence and awareness that not only benefits you but also positively impacts the children in your care. Simple practices such as mindful breathing, body scans, and guided imagery can help you ground yourself, making it easier to respond to emotional triggers with clarity and compassion.

One effective technique is mindful breathing, which involves focusing your attention on your breath. Take a moment to pause and breathe deeply, inhaling through your nose and exhaling through your mouth. This practice can be particularly useful during stressful moments, allowing you to regain composure and approach challenges with a calm mindset. Encourage your children to join you in this practice, helping them develop their own coping mechanisms for managing stress and emotional upheaval.

Another beneficial mindfulness practice is the body scan, which encourages awareness of physical sensations and emotional states. Set aside a few minutes each day to mentally scan your body from head to toe, noticing areas of tension or discomfort. This technique fosters a deeper connection to your own emotional triggers and can help you model self-awareness for the children you care for. By sharing your experiences with them, you create a safe space for discussion about feelings, encouraging them to express their emotions constructively.

Incorporating gratitude into your daily routine is another powerful mindfulness technique. Take a moment each day to reflect on three things you are grateful for, whether they are small moments of joy or significant achievements. This practice can shift your focus from stressors to positive aspects of your life, enhancing your overall emotional resilience. Sharing this practice with the children in your care fosters a culture of appreciation, helping them build a positive outlook and resilience in the face of their own challenges.

Lastly, consider establishing a daily mindfulness ritual, such as a short meditation or a nature walk, that you can share with your children. These rituals not only provide a structured time for mindfulness but also strengthen your bond with the children. As you practice mindfulness together, you create a supportive environment where emotional triggers can be addressed openly and constructively. By incorporating these techniques into your daily life, you not only promote your own well-being but also equip the children in your care with valuable tools for their emotional development.

Incorporating Mindfulness into Child Interaction

Incorporating mindfulness into interactions with children can significantly enhance the quality of caregiving, especially for surrogate parents, foster parents, and step-parents. Mindfulness, the practice of being present and fully engaged in the moment, allows caregivers to approach their interactions with a grounded perspective. This practice not only helps caregivers manage their own emotional triggers but also creates a nurturing environment where children can thrive. By fostering a mindful approach, caregivers can build stronger connections with their children, encouraging open communication and emotional resilience.

To begin integrating mindfulness into child interaction, caregivers can start with simple practices that promote awareness. For instance, taking a few deep breaths before engaging with a child can help center the caregiver's thoughts and emotions. This moment of pause allows caregivers to let go of any distractions or stressors, enabling them to be fully present. When caregivers are mindful, they model emotional regulation for their children, teaching them how to respond thoughtfully rather than react impulsively. This foundational practice can foster a sense of safety and security, crucial for children who may have experienced instability in their lives.

In addition to personal mindfulness practices, caregivers can create mindful moments during their interactions with children. This can be achieved through activities such as mindful listening or shared storytelling, where caregivers focus entirely on the child's words, feelings, and non-verbal cues. Such practices encourage children to express themselves and feel heard, which is vital for their emotional development. By being fully attentive, caregivers not only validate the child's experiences but also cultivate an atmosphere of trust. This emotional connection can serve as a protective factor against many psychological triggers that may arise in caregiving situations.

Mindfulness can also be woven into daily routines, transforming ordinary moments into opportunities for connection. For example, during mealtime, caregivers can practice gratitude by acknowledging the food and the effort that went into preparing it, encouraging children to do the same. This practice not only teaches appreciation but also enhances the mindfulness of the moment, allowing both the caregiver and the child to engage fully. By incorporating mindfulness into everyday activities, caregivers help children understand the importance of being present, which can lead to the development of their own coping mechanisms for stress.

Finally, caregivers can benefit from training programs focused on emotional awareness and mindfulness techniques. These programs can provide valuable strategies for managing emotional triggers and building resilience in children. By participating in such trainings, caregivers can deepen their understanding of mindfulness and equip themselves with practical tools for implementing these practices in their interactions. The development of a supportive community through these programs also fosters collaboration among parents and caregivers, enhancing their ability to navigate challenges together. As caregivers embrace mindfulness, they not only enrich their relationships with their children but also contribute to their overall emotional well-being and resilience.

6

Developing Coping Mechanisms for Caregivers

Recognizing Signs of Caregiver Stress

Recognizing signs of caregiver stress is crucial for surrogate parents, foster parents, and step-parents. Caregiving can be emotionally demanding, often leading to feelings of overwhelm and exhaustion. Understanding these signs is the first step toward addressing them effectively. This awareness not only benefits the caregiver but also enhances the well-being of the children in their care. By acknowledging stress, caregivers can take proactive measures to manage their emotional triggers and create a healthier environment for both themselves and the children they nurture.

One of the most common signs of caregiver stress is emotional fatigue. Caregivers may find themselves feeling irritable, anxious, or sad more often than usual. This emotional toll can negatively impact their ability to connect with the children in their care, potentially leading to misunderstandings or conflicts. It is essential for caregivers to check in with themselves regularly. Simple self-reflection can reveal whether feelings of frustration or sadness are becoming persistent, indicating the need for self-care and support.

Physical symptoms can also manifest as a result of caregiver stress. Caregivers might experience headaches, fatigue, or changes in appetite and sleep patterns. These physical signs are often the body's way of signaling that it is under strain. Recognizing these symptoms can prompt caregivers to take immediate action, such as seeking medical advice, engaging in physical activities, or practicing mindfulness techniques. Incorporating regular exercise and healthy eating can significantly enhance a caregiver's resilience and ability to cope with stress.

Social withdrawal is another indicator of caregiver stress that should not be overlooked. Caregivers may isolate themselves from friends and family, feeling that they cannot share their burdens or concerns. This isolation can exacerbate feelings of loneliness and anxiety. Encouraging caregivers to maintain social connections is vital. Support groups, whether in-person or online, can provide a safe space to share experiences and gain insight from others facing similar challenges. Building a network of support fosters resilience and helps caregivers feel less alone in their journey.

Ultimately, recognizing caregiver stress is about cultivating self-awareness and taking proactive steps toward self-care. Caregivers should remind themselves that they are not alone in this journey. By identifying the signs of stress, they can implement strategies to manage their emotional triggers, improve their well-being, and create a nurturing environment for the children they care for. Embracing mindfulness practices and developing coping mechanisms will not only enhance their resilience but also model healthy emotional management for the children, fostering a positive cycle of emotional well-being in the family dynamic.

Self-Care Strategies for Emotional Well-Being

Self-care is a vital aspect of maintaining emotional well-being, especially for surrogate parents, foster parents, and step-parents who often face unique challenges. These caregivers frequently encounter situations that can trigger intense emotional responses, whether due to past experiences or the complexity of their caregiving roles. By implementing effective self-care strategies, caregivers can cultivate a resilient mindset that not only benefits themselves but also positively impacts the children in their care. Embracing self-care is not a luxury; it is an essential practice that empowers caregivers to thrive amidst the demands of their responsibilities.

One powerful strategy for emotional well-being is establishing a routine that prioritizes personal time. Carving out moments for self-reflection, hobbies, or relaxation can significantly enhance emotional resilience. Caregivers should consider scheduling regular breaks, even if they are brief, to engage in activities that bring joy and fulfillment. Whether it's reading a book, taking a walk in nature, or practicing a favorite hobby, these moments of self-care can recharge emotional batteries and provide a necessary escape from caregiving stresses.

Mindfulness practices are another effective tool for managing emotional triggers. By incorporating mindfulness into daily routines, caregivers can develop greater awareness of their emotions and reactions. Techniques such as deep breathing, meditation, or mindful observation can help caregivers stay grounded during challenging moments. This heightened awareness allows for a more measured response to emotional triggers, fostering a sense of calm that can be communicated to the children. Practicing mindfulness not only benefits caregivers but also models healthy emotional regulation for the children they care for.

Building a support network is crucial for emotional well-being. Caregivers should seek connections with others who understand their unique challenges, whether through support groups, online forums, or friendships with other caregivers. Sharing experiences and strategies can provide validation and reduce feelings of isolation. In addition, these connections can be a source of encouragement and inspiration, reminding caregivers that they are not alone in their journey. A strong support network can be an invaluable resource for navigating the ups and downs of caregiving.

Finally, developing coping mechanisms is essential for managing the emotional landscape of caregiving. Caregivers can benefit from identifying specific strategies that work for them when faced with triggering situations. This might include journaling to process emotions, utilizing stress-relief techniques like exercise or art, or simply taking a moment to step away and regroup. By equipping themselves with effective coping tools, caregivers can respond to challenges with greater resilience and clarity. The journey of caregiving is undoubtedly demanding, but with consistent self-care practices, caregivers can foster their own emotional well-being while creating a nurturing environment for the children they love.

Building a Support Network

Building a support network is vital for surrogate parents, foster parents, and step-parents navigating the emotional complexities of child care. Establishing connections with others in similar situations can create a sense of belonging and understanding. When you share your experiences, challenges, and triumphs with those who truly comprehend your journey, it not only fosters emotional well-being but also equips you with valuable insights and coping strategies. These relationships can serve as a lifeline during difficult moments, reminding you that you are not alone in your caregiving role.

To successfully build this network, start by seeking out local or online support groups specifically designed for caregivers. These groups often provide a safe space for open discussions, allowing you to express your feelings and learn from others' experiences. Engaging with fellow caregivers can reveal common emotional triggers and suggest effective techniques for managing them. Whether it's through organized meetings, social media platforms, or dedicated forums, these connections can enhance your resilience and help cultivate a positive atmosphere for both you and the children in your care.

In addition to support groups, consider forming personal connections with friends and family who can offer emotional support. Sharing your journey with trusted individuals can provide a fresh perspective and practical advice. Don't hesitate to reach out to those who have experience in child care, as their insights may be incredibly beneficial. These relationships can also serve as informal mentors, guiding you through challenging situations and providing reassurance when you need it most.

Another effective way to build a support network is by collaborating with educators and professionals in your community. Engaging with teachers, counselors, and child psychologists can deepen your understanding of emotional triggers and enhance your strategies for coping. Many schools and community centers offer training programs focused on emotional awareness and resilience-building techniques. Participating in these programs not only expands your knowledge but also connects you with others committed to fostering a nurturing environment for children.

Ultimately, a robust support network cultivates resilience not just for caregivers but also for the children in their care. By sharing experiences and strategies, you foster an environment where emotional triggers are acknowledged and addressed together. This collaborative spirit enhances emotional stability, equipping both caregivers and children with the tools they need to navigate challenges. Remember, building a strong support network takes time and effort, but the rewards in emotional well-being and effective caregiving are immeasurable.

7

Training Programs on Emotional Awareness

Importance of Emotional Awareness in Child Care

Emotional awareness is a cornerstone of effective child care, particularly for surrogate parents, foster parents, and step-parents navigating complex family dynamics. Understanding the emotional landscape of both the caregiver and the child can significantly enhance the caregiving experience. When caregivers are attuned to their own emotions, they can better recognize and respond to the emotional triggers of the children in their care. This heightened awareness fosters a nurturing environment where children feel safe to express their feelings, which is crucial for their development and well-being.

Recognizing emotional triggers is essential for caregivers, as it allows them to respond thoughtfully rather than react impulsively. Children often communicate their needs and emotions through behavior, which can sometimes be challenging to interpret. By cultivating emotional awareness, caregivers can differentiate between a child's need for connection, attention, or independence. This understanding enables them to approach situations with empathy and patience, thereby reducing the likelihood of conflict and promoting a more harmonious home environment.

Building resilience in children is another vital aspect of emotional awareness in child care. When caregivers model emotional awareness—acknowledging their feelings and demonstrating healthy coping strategies—they provide children with valuable tools to navigate their own emotions. This modeling creates an environment where children learn to express their feelings constructively and develop resilience in the face of challenges. By fostering open dialogues about emotions, caregivers empower children to articulate their thoughts and feelings, ultimately supporting their emotional growth.

Mindfulness practices play a significant role in enhancing emotional awareness for both caregivers and children. By engaging in mindfulness techniques, caregivers can cultivate a sense of presence and clarity, enabling them to respond more effectively to the emotional needs of their children. Simple practices such as deep breathing, meditation, or mindful listening can transform stressful situations into opportunities for connection and understanding. When caregivers prioritize mindfulness, they not only improve their own emotional regulation but also create a calmer atmosphere for children to thrive.

Finally, training programs focused on emotional awareness can equip caregivers with the skills and knowledge needed to manage emotional triggers effectively. These programs can provide practical strategies for recognizing and addressing emotional challenges, enhancing both caregiver and child well-being. Collaborative techniques involving communication and teamwork between caregivers and children can further strengthen relationships, fostering a supportive environment that encourages growth and healing. By prioritizing emotional awareness, caregivers set the stage for a nurturing and resilient family dynamic, ultimately benefiting everyone involved.

Overview of Effective Training Programs

Effective training programs are essential for surrogate parents, foster parents, and step-parents seeking to navigate the complexities of emotional triggers in child care. These programs provide caregivers with the knowledge and skills necessary to recognize and address their own emotional responses, as well as those of the children in their care. By focusing on emotional awareness, caregivers can create a nurturing environment that promotes healing, resilience, and positive development. Understanding the foundational elements of effective training programs can empower caregivers to foster healthier relationships with children.

An effective training program begins with a strong emphasis on emotional awareness. Caregivers must learn to identify their own emotional triggers and understand how these feelings can impact their interactions with children. This self-awareness is crucial in preventing negative emotional responses that can arise in challenging situations. Training programs should incorporate strategies that help caregivers reflect on their emotional experiences, enabling them to respond thoughtfully rather than react impulsively. As a result, caregivers can model emotional regulation for the children they support, reinforcing the importance of managing feelings constructively.

Building resilience in children is another key component of effective training programs. Caregivers can learn techniques to help children develop coping mechanisms that equip them to face challenges and setbacks. Programs should include practical exercises and activities that promote problem-solving skills, emotional expression, and positive self-talk. By providing children with tools to navigate their emotional landscapes, caregivers can foster a sense of agency and confidence. This not only benefits the children but also enhances the caregivers' ability to support them effectively.

Mindfulness practices are increasingly recognized as valuable tools for caregivers in managing their own emotional triggers. Training programs that incorporate mindfulness techniques can help caregivers cultivate a sense of calm and presence, allowing them to respond to stressful situations with clarity and compassion. Simple practices such as deep breathing, meditation, and mindful observation can significantly reduce anxiety and enhance emotional well-being. By integrating mindfulness into their daily routines, caregivers can create a more peaceful environment for both themselves and the children they care for.

Collaboration among caregivers is vital for creating a supportive network that enhances the effectiveness of training programs. Encouraging open communication and sharing experiences can foster a sense of community among surrogate parents, foster parents, and step-parents. Training programs should facilitate opportunities for caregivers to connect, share strategies, and learn from one another. Through collaborative techniques, caregivers can develop a deeper understanding of their shared challenges and successes, ultimately leading to improved outcomes for the children in their care. This sense of camaraderie not only bolsters individual resilience but also strengthens the collective ability to support children through their emotional journeys.

Implementing Training in Daily Practice

Implementing training in daily practice is essential for surrogate parents, foster parents, and step-parents to effectively support the emotional development of the children in their care. The emotional triggers that children may exhibit can often be overwhelming, but by embedding training techniques into everyday routines, caregivers can create a nurturing environment that promotes healing and resilience. This approach not only benefits the children but also fosters the personal growth of caregivers, equipping them with the tools needed to navigate challenging situations with confidence and compassion.

To begin, it is crucial for caregivers to identify specific emotional triggers that may arise in their daily interactions with children. Developing a keen awareness of these triggers will enable caregivers to respond thoughtfully rather than reactively. This can be achieved through reflective practices such as journaling or engaging in discussions with peers or mentors. By regularly assessing their emotional responses and understanding the context behind them, caregivers can create a proactive strategy to manage these triggers effectively. Incorporating mindfulness techniques, such as deep breathing exercises or grounding practices, can help caregivers maintain their emotional balance when faced with challenging behaviors.

Furthermore, caregivers can cultivate resilience in children by employing consistent training techniques that reinforce positive behavior and emotional regulation. Techniques such as role-playing difficult scenarios or practicing problem-solving skills can empower children to understand their emotions and respond constructively. By integrating these activities into daily routines, caregivers not only provide children with practical skills but also model healthy emotional expression. Establishing a supportive atmosphere where children feel safe to share their feelings will encourage open communication, fostering deeper connections between caregivers and children.

Training programs specifically designed for emotional awareness can greatly enhance a caregiver's ability to implement these practices. Attending workshops or online courses can provide valuable insights into understanding emotional triggers and developing coping mechanisms. Collaborating with educators and mental health professionals can also enrich caregivers' knowledge and expand their toolkit. By networking with other caregivers, surrogate parents, and step-parents, individuals can share experiences and strategies that have proven effective, creating a community of support and ongoing learning.

Lastly, maintaining a consistent commitment to implementing training in daily practice is vital for long-term success. Caregivers should set realistic goals for their own emotional growth alongside their children's development. Regularly revisiting training methods and adapting them to meet the evolving needs of the child will ensure a dynamic and responsive caregiving approach. Embracing this journey with patience and persistence will not only enhance the emotional well-being of the children but also empower caregivers to thrive in their roles, transforming challenges into opportunities for growth and connection.

8

Collaborative Techniques

Building Strong Partnerships with Parents

Building strong partnerships with parents is essential for surrogate parents, foster parents, and step-parents who aim to create a nurturing environment for the children in their care. Collaborating with biological parents, when possible, fosters a sense of continuity for the child and promotes a unified approach to their emotional and developmental needs. Establishing open lines of communication is crucial; regular check-ins, whether through phone calls, emails, or face-to-face meetings, can help build rapport and trust. By sharing insights about the child's progress and challenges, caregivers can empower parents to be active participants in their child's life, which can significantly enhance the child's emotional well-being.

Understanding the emotional triggers that parents may face is equally important. Many parents come from a variety of backgrounds and experiences that shape their responses to parenting situations. Through empathetic listening, caregivers can gain insight into these triggers and work collaboratively to develop strategies that address them. For instance, if a parent struggles with anxiety during transitions, caregivers can create supportive routines that ease these moments, allowing both the child and the parent to feel more secure. By recognizing and validating these feelings, caregivers can help parents move past their psychological triggers, fostering a more positive partnership.

Effective partnerships also involve setting mutual goals and expectations. Caregivers should invite parents to participate in developing consistent behavioral expectations and routines that align between the home and the caregiving environment. This collaborative goal-setting can include discussing discipline strategies, communication methods, and emotional support techniques. When parents and caregivers are on the same page, it not only helps to reinforce the child's learning and emotional growth but also strengthens the bond between all adults involved in the child's life. These shared objectives can lead to a more harmonious atmosphere, benefiting everyone.

Mindfulness practices can serve as a foundation for building these partnerships. Encouraging parents to engage in mindfulness techniques can help them manage their emotional responses, ultimately benefiting their interactions with their children. Simple practices, such as breathing exercises or reflective journaling, can provide parents with tools to enhance their emotional regulation. By sharing these techniques, caregivers can model the importance of self-awareness and emotional health, fostering a culture of resilience not only for the children but for the parents as well.

Continuous training and support for caregivers and parents are vital for maintaining strong partnerships. Workshops and training programs focused on emotional awareness can enhance understanding and improve communication strategies. These sessions can provide valuable resources for both caregivers and parents, equipping them with coping mechanisms and collaborative techniques that benefit everyone involved. By investing in their own growth and development, caregivers demonstrate a commitment to creating a supportive environment that prioritizes the emotional well-being of the child, thereby reinforcing a strong, effective partnership with parents.

Effective Communication Strategies

Effective communication is a cornerstone in fostering strong relationships between caregivers and children, especially in the context of navigating emotional triggers. Surrogate parents, foster parents, and step-parents often face unique challenges that can lead to misunderstandings and heightened emotions. By adopting effective communication strategies, caregivers can create a supportive environment that promotes emotional well-being for both themselves and the children in their care. This approach not only enhances trust but also facilitates a deeper understanding of the emotional needs of children, allowing for more effective responses to their triggers.

One essential strategy is active listening. This involves giving full attention to the child, acknowledging their feelings, and responding thoughtfully. By practicing active listening, caregivers can validate a child's emotions, making them feel heard and understood. This validation can significantly alleviate feelings of frustration or anger that often arise from emotional triggers. Additionally, caregivers should mirror the child's emotions, which fosters empathy and encourages the child to express themselves more openly. When children feel that their emotions are recognized, they are more likely to share their thoughts and concerns, leading to healthier communication patterns.

Another effective strategy is the use of "I" statements. These statements allow caregivers to express their feelings and needs without placing blame or causing defensiveness in the child. For instance, instead of saying, "You never listen to me," a caregiver might say, "I feel upset when I don't feel heard." This approach not only models emotional expression but also encourages children to articulate their feelings and needs more clearly. By fostering an environment where expressing emotions is safe, caregivers can help children learn to manage their own emotional triggers, ultimately building resilience.

In addition to verbal communication, nonverbal cues play a significant role in how messages are received. Caregivers should be mindful of their body language, facial expressions, and tone of voice. Maintaining eye contact, using an open posture, and speaking in a calm, reassuring tone can convey support and understanding. These nonverbal signals can reinforce the caregiver's commitment to creating a safe space for emotional expression. By being attuned to both verbal and nonverbal communication, caregivers can better navigate complex emotional situations and provide the guidance that children need.

Lastly, fostering a collaborative atmosphere is crucial. Caregivers should encourage children to participate in discussions about their feelings and experiences. By inviting children to share their thoughts, caregivers empower them to take ownership of their emotional journeys. Collaborative techniques can involve brainstorming solutions together, establishing family rules, or creating a shared journal where feelings can be expressed. This inclusive approach not only strengthens the caregiver-child bond but also equips children with vital coping mechanisms for managing their emotional triggers, ultimately leading to healthier outcomes in their emotional development.

Team Approaches to Child Development

Team approaches to child development emphasize the importance of collaboration among caregivers, educators, and professionals to create a nurturing environment that fosters emotional growth and resilience in children. For surrogate parents, foster parents, and step-parents, understanding the dynamics of a team approach can significantly enhance the quality of care provided to children. Through open communication, shared goals, and mutual support, caregivers can work together to address emotional triggers and promote healthy development in children, ensuring that they feel secure and valued.

One of the key aspects of a successful team approach is the establishment of clear roles and responsibilities. Each caregiver brings unique strengths and perspectives to the table, and recognizing these can lead to more effective strategies for managing emotional triggers. By identifying individual capabilities and areas of expertise, caregivers can create a supportive network where everyone feels empowered to contribute. This collaborative spirit not only fosters a sense of community but also reinforces the idea that caring for a child is a shared responsibility, ultimately benefiting the child's emotional well-being.

Communication is vital in a team approach. Regular meetings and open discussions allow caregivers to share insights, challenges, and successes. This transparency cultivates trust and encourages a culture of feedback, where caregivers can learn from one another's experiences. By actively listening and engaging in constructive dialogue, caregivers can develop a deeper understanding of each child's needs and create tailored strategies to help them navigate their emotional landscapes. This process not only aids in managing triggers but also teaches children the value of empathy and collaboration.

Building resilience in children requires consistent and coordinated efforts from all caregivers involved. Team approaches enable caregivers to implement cohesive strategies that reinforce positive behaviors and coping mechanisms. By working together to set achievable goals and celebrate milestones, caregivers can instill a sense of accomplishment in children. This collective effort helps children develop the confidence to face challenges and fosters a growth mindset, equipping them with the tools necessary to manage their emotions effectively.

Mindfulness practices can also be integrated into team approaches, benefiting both caregivers and children. By incorporating mindfulness techniques into daily routines, caregivers can model emotional awareness and self-regulation. These practices not only help caregivers manage their own emotional triggers but also teach children valuable skills for coping with stress and anxiety. When caregivers are mindful of their own responses, they create a calm and supportive environment that encourages children to express their feelings openly. Ultimately, a team approach to child development nurtures resilience, promotes emotional awareness, and strengthens the bonds between caregivers and children, paving the way for a brighter future.

9

Creating a Supportive Environment

Designing Safe Spaces for Emotional Expression

Creating safe spaces for emotional expression is essential for fostering resilience in children, especially in the context of surrogate parenting, foster care, and blended families. As caregivers, understanding the importance of these spaces can significantly impact a child's ability to process their emotions and build healthy coping mechanisms. A safe emotional environment encourages children to express their feelings openly, knowing they will be met with understanding and support. This foundation is crucial for helping them navigate their psychological triggers and emotional challenges.

To design an effective safe space, start by establishing clear and consistent routines that promote predictability. Children thrive in environments where they know what to expect. By integrating regular check-ins and designated times for open dialogue, caregivers can create a rhythm that allows children to feel secure. These routines can include family meetings, storytelling sessions, or simple daily reflections where everyone shares their thoughts and feelings. This structure not only aids emotional expression but also strengthens the bond between caregivers and children.

In addition to routines, the physical environment plays a vital role in creating a safe space. Consider designating a specific area in your home as an emotional sanctuary. This space should be inviting and comfortable, filled with items that promote relaxation, such as soft seating, calming colors, and sensory toys. Incorporating elements like art supplies or journals can encourage children to express their emotions through creativity. Providing a visually and tactilely appealing environment can help children feel more at ease when discussing their feelings.

Another critical aspect of designing safe spaces is active listening. Caregivers should practice being fully present when children share their emotions, responding without judgment or interruption. This approach fosters a sense of validation and respect for their feelings. Techniques such as reflective listening, where caregivers paraphrase what the child has said, can help clarify emotions and demonstrate that their feelings are heard and understood. By modeling empathetic communication, caregivers can empower children to articulate their emotions more effectively.

Finally, incorporating mindfulness practices into the safe space can enhance emotional expression and regulation. Simple techniques such as breathing exercises, guided imagery, or mindfulness games can help children center themselves before engaging in emotional discussions. These practices not only provide tools for immediate emotional management but also instill long-term coping strategies. Encouraging caregivers to share these practices with their children can strengthen their relationship and foster an atmosphere of emotional safety, ultimately leading to healthier emotional development.

Encouraging Open Dialogue

Encouraging open dialogue is essential for creating a nurturing environment where children feel safe to express their feelings and thoughts. As surrogate parents, foster parents, and step-parents, you have the unique opportunity to foster a sense of trust and security that encourages children to communicate openly. By actively listening and validating their emotions, you can help them navigate their psychological triggers, leading to healthier interactions and emotional resilience. When children know that their voices matter, they are more likely to share their experiences, which can be a vital step in understanding and addressing their emotional needs.

Creating an environment that promotes open dialogue starts with establishing routines and practices that prioritize communication. Regular family meetings can be an effective way to set aside time for everyone to share their thoughts and feelings. During these gatherings, encourage each child to express themselves without fear of judgment. This routine helps normalize conversations about emotions and allows children to witness how emotional triggers can be discussed openly, fostering a culture of honesty and support. By modeling this behavior, you can teach children that discussing their feelings is a strength, not a vulnerability.

In addition to structured conversations, informal moments can also serve as opportunities for dialogue. Simple activities, such as cooking together or going for a walk, can create a relaxed atmosphere where children may feel more comfortable sharing their thoughts. Pay attention to nonverbal cues and encourage children to articulate what they are experiencing. By being present and attentive, you can help them understand their feelings better, reinforcing the idea that it's okay to talk about what they're going through. These moments can be crucial in building resilience, as children learn to recognize and manage their emotional triggers in real-time.

As caregivers, it's also important to practice self-awareness and emotional regulation. Your responses to children's emotional expressions set the tone for open dialogue. When caregivers demonstrate patience and understanding, children are more likely to reciprocate with honesty. Share your feelings and experiences with age-appropriate language, allowing them to see that everyone has emotions that can be managed and discussed. This transparency fosters a sense of connection and normalizes the experience of navigating emotional challenges together.

Finally, consider incorporating mindfulness practices into your daily routines. Mindfulness can enhance emotional awareness and provide tools for both caregivers and children to manage triggers effectively. Techniques such as deep breathing, meditation, or simply taking a moment to reflect can create a shared understanding of emotional states. Encourage children to express their feelings as they arise, reinforcing that open dialogue is an ongoing process. As you cultivate this practice together, you not only strengthen your bond but also empower children with the skills they need to navigate their emotional landscapes, leading to lasting resilience and harmony in your home.

Celebrating Emotional Milestones

Celebrating emotional milestones is a vital aspect of nurturing the psychological well-being of children in your care. As surrogate parents, foster parents, and step-parents, you play a crucial role in helping children navigate their emotional landscapes. Recognizing and celebrating these milestones not only validates their feelings but also promotes resilience. Each small victory, whether it's expressing a difficult emotion or overcoming a fear, deserves acknowledgment. By celebrating these moments, you reinforce the idea that emotional growth is a journey worth recognizing, thereby fostering a supportive environment for the child.

One effective way to celebrate these milestones is through the use of positive reinforcement. When a child articulates their feelings or successfully copes with a challenging situation, acknowledging their effort can significantly boost their confidence. Consider creating a "milestone chart" where you can document these achievements together. Each time they reach a new milestone, celebrate with a special activity or treat. This approach not only makes the child feel appreciated but also encourages them to continue exploring their emotions in a healthy way.

Incorporating mindfulness practices into your routine can also enhance the celebration of emotional milestones. Mindfulness encourages both caregivers and children to be present and aware of their emotions without judgment. After a significant emotional breakthrough, take time to reflect together. Engage in calming activities such as deep breathing exercises or guided imagery, allowing the child to process their feelings in a safe space. This not only solidifies the importance of the milestone but also teaches them valuable coping mechanisms that will serve them well in the future.

Collaboration with other caregivers and educators can amplify the celebration of these milestones. Sharing experiences and strategies with other adults involved in the child's life creates a unified approach to emotional support. Organize workshops or informal gatherings where caregivers can exchange stories, discuss emotional triggers, and celebrate each child's progress together. This collective effort not only strengthens the support network for the child but also cultivates a community that values emotional awareness and growth.

Ultimately, celebrating emotional milestones sets the stage for long-term resilience and emotional intelligence. As caregivers, your role extends beyond day-to-day care; you are instrumental in helping children build a solid foundation for their emotional future. By consistently recognizing and celebrating their achievements, you empower them to face challenges with confidence and develop healthy coping strategies. Embrace these moments, for they are not just milestones; they are stepping stones on the path to emotional well-being.

10

Moving Forward: Your Journey as a Caregiver

Setting Goals for Personal Growth

Setting goals for personal growth is an essential step for surrogate parents, foster parents, and step-parents who aspire to create a nurturing environment for the children in their care. By establishing clear and achievable goals, caregivers can not only enhance their own emotional resilience but also model positive behavior for the children they support. This process begins with self-reflection, where caregivers assess their strengths, weaknesses, and emotional triggers. Identifying these areas allows for targeted goal setting that can lead to meaningful personal development and improved caregiving practices.

Once self-awareness is established, it's important to set specific, measurable, achievable, relevant, and time-bound (SMART) goals. For instance, a caregiver might aim to practice mindfulness for ten minutes a day to better manage stress and emotional triggers. By breaking down larger aspirations into manageable tasks, caregivers can track their progress and celebrate small victories. This not only boosts their confidence but also reinforces the importance of setting goals to the children they care for, demonstrating that personal growth is a continuous journey.

In developing these goals, caregivers should consider the emotional needs of the children they support. Setting goals such as implementing daily check-ins with each child can foster open communication and trust. By incorporating the emotional well-being of the children into their own personal growth objectives, caregivers create a harmonious environment that promotes healing and resilience. This collaborative approach ensures that both caregivers and children benefit from the growth process, strengthening their bond and enhancing overall family dynamics.

Moreover, caregivers should seek out training programs and resources that align with their goals. Workshops focused on emotional awareness, resilience-building strategies, and mindfulness practices can provide valuable tools and techniques. By investing in their education and personal development, caregivers are better equipped to handle emotional triggers and model healthy coping mechanisms for the children in their care. Engaging in these opportunities allows for continuous learning and adaptation, which is crucial in the ever-evolving landscape of child care.

Lastly, accountability plays a vital role in achieving personal growth goals. Caregivers can benefit from forming support networks with other surrogate, foster, and step-parents. Sharing experiences, challenges, and successes fosters a sense of community and mutual encouragement. By holding each other accountable, caregivers can stay motivated and committed to their personal growth journey. This collaborative spirit not only enhances individual resilience but also instills a sense of stability and security for the children, ensuring that everyone involved thrives in a nurturing and supportive environment.

Continuous Learning and Adaptation

Continuous learning and adaptation are essential components of effective caregiving, particularly for surrogate parents, foster parents, and step-parents navigating the complexities of emotional triggers in child care. As caregivers, understanding that every child is unique, with their own set of experiences and emotional responses, is vital. Embracing a mindset of continuous learning allows caregivers to stay open to new strategies and insights that can enhance their emotional awareness and responsiveness. By actively seeking out knowledge and training, caregivers can better equip themselves to manage their own emotional triggers while fostering a supportive environment for the children in their care.

One of the most powerful tools in this journey is the practice of mindfulness. Mindfulness encourages caregivers to remain present and attuned to their own feelings and those of the children they care for. By incorporating mindfulness practices into daily routines, caregivers can develop a greater awareness of emotional triggers as they arise. Techniques such as deep breathing, meditation, and reflective journaling can help caregivers process their emotions and respond more thoughtfully to challenging situations. This not only aids in personal resilience but also models emotional regulation for children, teaching them valuable coping mechanisms that they can carry into their own lives.

In addition to mindfulness, caregivers can benefit from actively seeking out training programs focused on emotional awareness and resilience-building. Many organizations offer workshops and resources tailored to the specific needs of caregivers, helping them understand the psychological triggers that may affect their interactions with children. These programs often provide practical strategies for managing emotional responses and developing healthier communication patterns. By investing time in these educational opportunities, caregivers can enhance their skills and create a more nurturing environment that encourages emotional growth for both themselves and the children they care for.

Collaboration among caregivers and parents is another key aspect of continuous learning. Engaging in open dialogue about emotional challenges can foster a sense of community and shared understanding. Support groups, online forums, and local meetups can serve as platforms for caregivers to exchange experiences, strategies, and resources. This collaborative approach not only helps caregivers feel less isolated in their struggles but also allows them to learn from one another's successes and setbacks. By building a network of support, caregivers can adapt their practices in real-time, ensuring that they are responsive to the evolving needs of the children they serve.

Ultimately, continuous learning and adaptation are about embracing the journey of growth, both for caregivers and the children in their care. By committing to self-improvement and remaining open to new ideas, caregivers can cultivate a resilient environment that empowers children to navigate their own emotional landscapes. This ongoing process reinforces the importance of flexibility and understanding in caregiving, reminding us that each day presents an opportunity to learn, adapt, and thrive together. In doing so, caregivers not only enhance their own emotional well-being but also lay the groundwork for healthier, more resilient future generations.

Embracing the Caregiver Experience

Embracing the caregiver experience is a journey filled with unique challenges and profound rewards. As surrogate parents, foster parents, and step-parents, you are often stepping into roles that require you to navigate complex emotional landscapes, both for yourself and the children in your care. Understanding and embracing this experience is crucial in fostering a nurturing environment where both you and your children can thrive. Recognizing the emotional triggers that arise in caregiving allows you to take proactive steps towards managing them, enabling you to create a stable and supportive atmosphere that promotes growth and healing.

The emotional triggers you may encounter can stem from various sources, including past experiences, societal pressures, or the specific needs of the children you care for. It's essential to acknowledge these triggers without judgment, as they are part of the caregiver's emotional landscape. One effective strategy is to practice mindfulness, which encourages you to stay present and grounded in the moment. By cultivating an awareness of your thoughts and feelings, you can better understand how they influence your reactions. This self-awareness not only helps you manage your emotional responses but also sets a powerful example for the children in your care, teaching them the value of recognizing and processing their emotions.

Building resilience in children is another vital aspect of the caregiver experience. When children feel safe and supported, they are more likely to develop coping mechanisms that will serve them throughout their lives. As caregivers, you can foster resilience by providing consistent emotional support, encouraging open communication, and validating their feelings. Incorporating activities that promote emotional expression, such as art or storytelling, can also help children learn to articulate their experiences, thus reducing the impact of emotional triggers. Remember that resilience is not just about overcoming challenges; it's about learning and growing from them, a lesson you can impart through your own experiences.

Developing coping mechanisms for yourself as a caregiver is equally important. Engage in self-care practices that nourish your well-being, such as establishing boundaries, seeking support from peers, or setting aside time for relaxation. These practices not only enhance your emotional health but also equip you with the tools to handle stress more effectively. Training programs focused on emotional awareness can also be beneficial, allowing you to deepen your understanding of your emotional landscape and develop strategies that work for you. Consider participating in workshops or support groups that emphasize collaboration and shared experiences, as these can provide valuable insights and foster connections with others who understand your journey.

Ultimately, embracing the caregiver experience means recognizing the interconnectedness of your emotions with those of the children in your care. By fostering a collaborative approach with other caregivers and educators, you create a network of support that benefits everyone involved. Share techniques and strategies that have worked for you, and be open to learning from others. This collaborative spirit not only enhances your own resilience but also creates a richer, more supportive environment for the children you nurture. Together, you can navigate the complexities of caregiving, transforming emotional triggers into opportunities for growth and connection.

www.ingramcontent.com/pod-product-compliance
Ingram Content Group UK Ltd.
Pitfield, Milton Keynes, MK11 3LW, UK
UKHW030816300125
454392UK00001B/1